An Introduction to Human Services